FREE THE BRAIN LOCK

S. Saradhadevi

RIGI PUBLICATION

FREE THE BRAIN LOCK

BY

S. Saradhadevi

Originally published in India

ISBN: 978-93-95773-22-5

Published by RIGI PUBLICATION

777, Street no.9, Krishna Nagar

Khanna-141401 (Punjab), India

Website: www.rigipublication.com

Email: info@rigipublication.com

Phone: +91-9357710014, +91-9465468291

TABLE OF CONTENT

EFFECTIVENESS OF SLEEP HYGIENE TO REDUCE INSOMNIA AMONG PERSONS WITH SUFFERING WITH OBSESSIVE COMPULSIVE DISORDER

SARADHADEVI.S
RESEARCH SCHOLAR

DR.V.HEMAVATHYSUPERVISOR
PRINCIPAL
SREE BALAJI COLLEGE OF NURSING
BHARATH INSTITUTE OF HIGHER EDUCATION AND RESEARCH

Abstract

Insomnia is a common problem among patients with obsessive-compulsive disorder and patients suffering from acute insomnia with psychiatric comorbidity are more likely to develop chronic insomnia without appropriate intervention. Here we report a case of obsessive-compulsive disorder with acute insomnia, successfully treated with early sleep psychiatric non-pharmacological intervention.Sleep is crucial to brain function and import formaintainig cognitive and emotional process. Insomnia and anxiety disorders are highly prevalent and are associated with significant impairment and disability. There is evidence thatinsomnia and anxiety disorders commonly co-occur, in addition to both being highly comorbid with major depressive disorder.Sleep hygiene has been incorporated into most psychological interventions for insomnia. Clinically, these instructions provide a good start for treatment.

Key words: Sleep, Insomnia, Obsession, compulsion

Introduction

Psychiatric disorders, such as neurotic disorders including OCD, are often associated with sleep disorders, especially insomnia, which is a crucial element in clinical practice.It is chronic inability to obtain the amount of sleep needed for optimal functioning and well- being. Behavioral interventions for insomnia include relaxation training, stimulus control therapy, sleep restriction therapy, sleep hygiene, paradoxical intention therapy, cognitive restructuring, and other approaches. These are briefly explained. Research indicates that behavioral interventions are efficacious, effective, and likely cost-effective treatments for insomnia that yield reliable, robust, and long-term benefits in adults of all ages. Detailed guidance is provided for the practical management of patients with insomnia.

Materials and Methods

Quantitative evaluative research approach was used to assess the effectiveness of sleephygiene to reduce insomnia among OCD Persons. Experimental research design was used for the study. The sample was alcohol dependence between the age group of 18 to above 60 years who fulfil the inclusion criteria. Probability simple random sampling technique was used.The tool consists of 3parts, demographic variables, insomnia severity index scale and interventions.

OBJECTIVES OF THE STUDY

1. To determine the pre and post assessment level of insomnia among persons sufferingwith obsessive compulsive disorder in study and control group
2. To compare pre and post assessment level insomnia among persons suffering withobsessive compulsive disorder in study and control group
3. To evaluate the effectiveness of sleep hygiene to reduce insomnia for personssuffering with obsessive compulsive disorder between study and control group.
4. To associate demographic variables with posttest level of scores in study group.

RESULTS

Table 1: PRETEST LEVEL OF INSOMNIA SCORE

Level of insomnia	Experiment		Control		Chi square test
	n	%	n	%	
No clinically significant insomnia	0	0.00%	0	0.00%	$\chi2=0.37$ P=0.54 (NS)
Sub threshold insomnia	1	6.67%	2	13.33%	
Moderate severity	14	93.33%	13	86.67%	
Severe	0	0.00%	0	0.00%	
Total	15	100.00%	15	100.00%	

(Fig 6) P>0.05 not significant   NS= not significant

Table no.2 compares the pretest level of insomniascore between Experiment and control group of persons suffering with obsessive compulsive disorder before intervention.Before Multi interventional approach, in Experimentgroup, 6.67% of themare having Sub threshold insomnialevel of score, 93.33% of them having Moderate severity level of score .In control group ,13.33% of themare having Sub threshold insomnia level of score, 86.67% of them having Moderate severity level of score . Statistically there is no significant difference between Experiment and control group. Level of insomnia score betweenExperiment and control group was calculated using chi-square test.

Table 2 POSTTEST LEVEL OF INSOMNIA SCORE

Level of insomnia	Experiment		Control		Chi square test
	n	%	n	%	
No clinically significant insomnia	0	0.00%	0	0.00%	**$\chi2=3.97$ P=0.05***
Sub threshold insomnia	7	46.67%	2	13.33%	

Moderate severity	8	53.33%	13	86.67%	**(S)**
Severe	0	0.00%	0	0.00%	
Total	15	100.00%	15	100.00%	

(Fig 8) ***P≤0.001very high significant S= significant

Table no.2 compares the post-test level of insomnia *score between Experiment and control group of* persons suffering with obsessive compulsive disorder before intervention.Before Multi interventional approach, in Experiment group, 46.67% of themare having Sub thresholdinsomnia level of score, 53.33% of them having Moderate severity level of score .In controlgroup ,13.33% of themare having Sub threshold insomnia level of score, 86.67% of them having Moderate severity level of score .

Statistically there is a significant difference between Experiment and control group. Level ofinsomnia score between Experiment and control group was calculated using chi-square test.

Level of Insomnia score between Experiment and control group

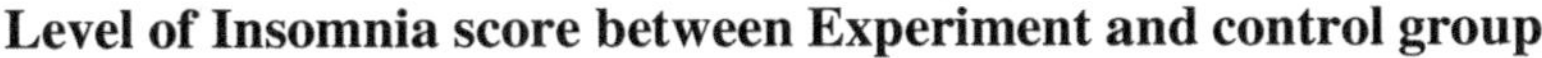

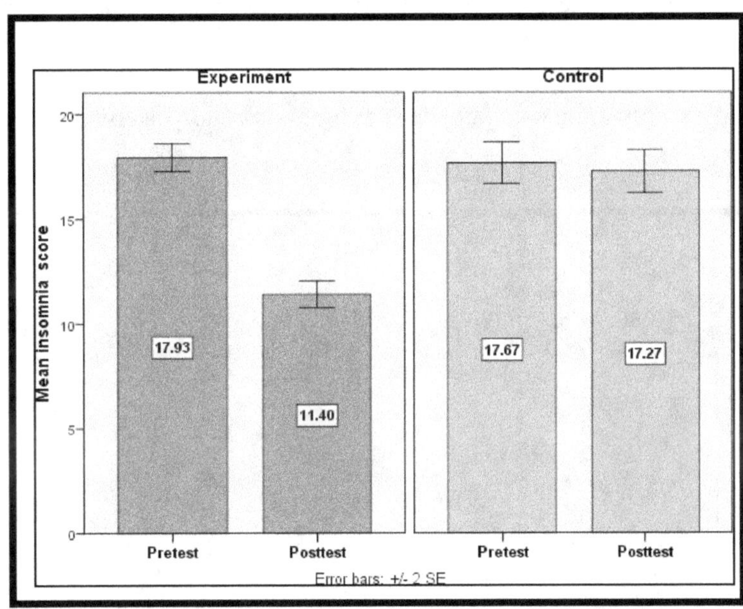

Table 3: COMPARISON OF PRETEST AND POSTTEST MEANINSOMNIA SCORE

Group		N	Mean	SD	Mean reduction score	Paired t-test
Experiment	Pre-test	15	17.93	1.28	6.53	**t=11.55 p=0.001*** (S)**
	Post-test	15	11.40	1.24		
Control	Pre-test	15	17.67	1.91	0.40	t=1.57 p=0.14 (NS)
	Post-test	15	17.27	1.00		

Considering Experiment group, in pretest they are having 17.93score and in posttest they arehaving 11.40 score, so the difference is 6.53 this difference is large and it is statistically significant.

Considering Control group, in pretest they are having 17.67 score and in posttest they are having 17.27score, so the difference is 0.40, this difference is small and it is not statisticallysignificant.

Statistical significance difference between pre-test and post-test was calculated using studentpaired t-test

Table 4: COMPARISON OF MEAN INSOMNIA SCORE BETWEENEXPERIMENT AND CONTROL GROUP

Group		N	Mean	SD	Mean difference score	Student independent t-test
Pretest	Experiment	15	17.93	1.28	0.26	t=0.45 p=0.66 (NS)
	Control	15	17.67	1.91		
Posttest	Experiment	15	11.40	1.24	5.87	**t=10.73 p=0.001*** (S)**
	Control	15	17.27	1.02		

Considering pretest,Experiment group are having 17.93score and in control they are having 17.67 score, so the difference is 0.93, this difference is small   and it is statistically notsignificant.

Considering posttest, Experiment group are having 11.40 score and in control group, they are having 17.07score, so the difference is 14.57, this difference is large and it is statistically significant.

Statistical significance difference between experiment and control was calculated using student independent t-test

Simple bar with 2 standard errordiagram compares the pretest and posttestInsomnia scoreamong Experiment and Control group

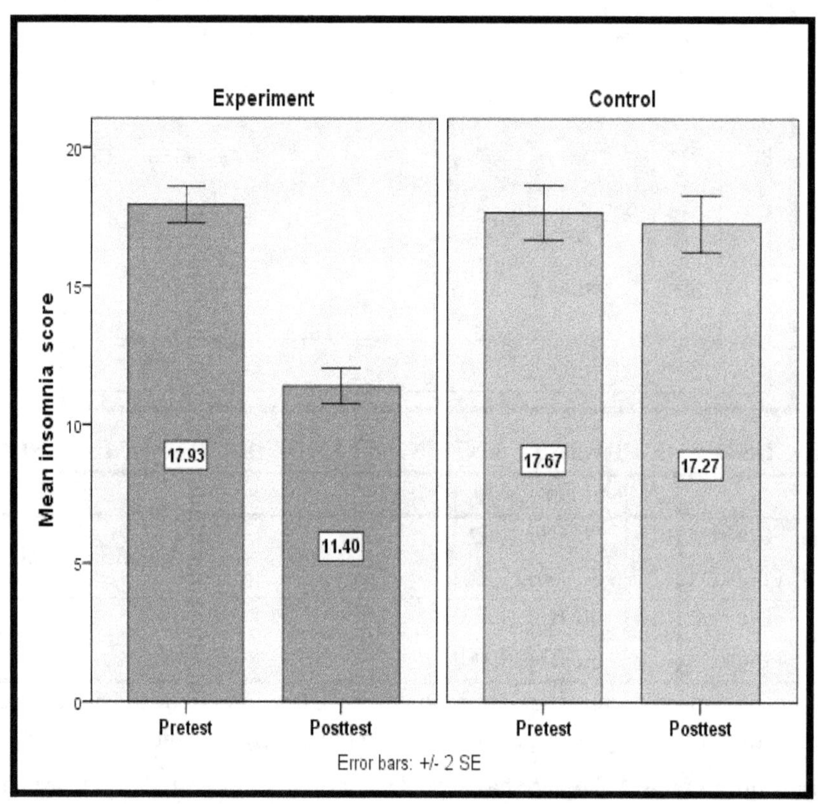

Table 5: EFFECTIVENESS OF MULTIINTERVENTIONAL APPROACH AND GENRALIZATION OF INSOMNIAREDUCTION SCORE

Group	Test	Maximum score	Mean score	Mean Difference of insomnia reduction score with 95% Confidence interval	Percentage Difference of insomnia reduction score with 95% Confidence interval
Experiment	Pretest	28	17.93	6.53(5.31 – 7.75)	23.32%(18.96% – 27.67%)
	Posttest	28	11.40		
Control	Pretest	28	17.67	0.40(-0.15 – 0.95)	1.42%(-0.54% – 3.39%)
	Posttest	28	17.27		

Table no 5 shows the effectiveness of effectiveness of multiinterventional approachoninsomnia.

Experiment group are reduced23.32% insomnascore whereas control group reducedonly3.39% of score.

Differences and generalization of insomnia reductionscore*betweenpretest and posttest scorewas calculated using and mean difference with 95% CI and proportion with 95% CI*

Table 6 : ASSOCIATION BETWEEN POSTTEST LEVEL OF INSOMNIA SCORE AND PERSONS DEMOGRAPHIC VARIBLES(Experiment group)

Demographic variables		Sub threshold insomnia		Moderate severity		n	Chi square test
		n	%		%		
AGE	31-40 years	4	50.00%	4	50.00%	8	$\chi2=0.07 p=0.78$(NS)
	41-50 years	3	42.86%	4	57.14%	7	
RELIGION	Hindu	3	20.00%	7	80.00%	10	$\chi2=0.83 p=0.36$(NS)
	Muslim/Christian	4	100.00%	1	0.00%	5	
TYPE OF FAMILY	Nuclear family	6	54.55%	5	45.45%	11	$\chi2=1.02 p=0.31$(NS)
	Joint family	1	25.00%	3	75.00%	4	
MARITAL STATUS	Married	7	46.67%	8	53.33%	15	$\chi2=0.00 p=1.00$(NS)
	Unmarried	0	0.00%	0	0.00%	0	
OCCUPATION	Cooley /Drivers	2	20.00%	8	80.00%	10	**$\chi2=5.65 p=0.01$**(S)
	Businessman/others	5	100.00%	0	0.00%	5	
SUPPORT	Family	7	63.64%	4	36.36%	11	**$\chi2=4.77 p=0.05$*(S)**

SYSTEM	Relatives	0	0.00%	4	100.00%	4	
DURATION OF	2- 3 hours	1	16.67%	5	83.33%	6	χ2=1.88p=0.17NS)
SLEP PER DAY	3- 4 hours	6	66.67%	3	33.33%	9	
SLEEP HABITS	Listing to music/others	1	16.67%	5	83.33%	6	χ2=2.88p=0.17(NS)
	Watching TV	6	66.67%	3	33.33%	9	

***p≤0.01 highly significant *p≤0.05 significant S=significant*

p>0.05 not significant NS= not significant

Table 6 shows the association between the post-test level of insomnia score and demographic variables of persons. businessman/others and family support persons are morebenefited than others. Statistical significance was assessed using Chi square test/Yates corrected chi square test.

Discussion

Psychological and behavioural therapies reliable changes in several sleep parameters with insomnia associated with medical and psychiatric disorders. sleep psychiatry (psychiatric therapeutic approach, both biologically and psychologically, based on sleep science) has gathered much attention worldwide. In this case, we attempted an early intervention in the vicious cycle of acute insomnia.

References:

1. Tenney NH, Schotte CK, Denys DA, Van Megen HJ, Westenberg HG. Assessment of DSM-IV personality disorders in obsessive–compulsive disorder: comparison of clinical diagnosis, self-report questionnaire, andsemi-structured interview. J Pers Disord. 2003;17:550–61

2. Ruscio AM, Stein DJ, Chiu WT, Kessler RC. The epidemiology of obsessive-compulsive disorder in the National Comorbidity Survey Replication. *Mol Psychiatry*. 2010;15(1):53–63.

3. Huppert JD, Simpson HB, Nissenson KJ, Liebowitz MR, Foa EB. Quality of life and functional impairment in obsessive-compulsive disorder. *Depress Anxiety*. 2009;26(1):39–45.

4. Visser HA, van Oppen P, van Megen HJ, et al. Obsessive-compulsive disorder. *J Affect Disord*. 2014;152– 154:169–174.

5. Eisen JL, Sibrava NJ, Boisseau CL, et al. Five-year course of obsessive-compulsive disorder. *J ClinPsychiatry*. 2013;74(3):233–239.

IJCRT.ORG **ISSN : 2320-2882**

INTERNATIONAL JOURNAL OF CREATIVE RESEARCH THOUGHTS (IJCRT)

An International Open Access, Peer-reviewed, Refereed Journal

EFFECTIVENESS OF PROGRESSIVE MUSCLE RELAXATION TECHNIQUE ON MENTALLY ILL PATIENTS

SARADHADEVI.S

Research Scholar

Sree Balaji College of Nursing

Bharath Institute of Higher Education and

ResearchDr.V.HEMAVATHY

SUPERVISOR

PRINCIPAL, SREE BALAJI COLLEGE OF NURSING, BIHER.

ABSTRACT:

Anxiety is a normal response to human experience and survival not unlike the flight, or hide response, humans need anxiety in order to act and to protect them from suffering. It is the result of unresolved trauma leaving the individual in a heightened physiological state if arousal in which certain experiences have the potential to reactivate the old trauma, as is often the case post traumatic stress. Sometimes anxiety results from a lack of, or inexperience at, knowing how to self-sooth and there are other psychological andemotional reasons for anxiety.

KEYWORDS: Progressive muscle,Relaxation,Mentally ill,Anxiety

OBJECTIVES

- ❑ To determine the pretest and post test level of anxiety among mentally ill patients in experimental andcontrol group.

- ❑ To determine the effectiveness of Progressive Muscle Relaxation Technique on anxiety among mentally ill patients.

To associate the post level of anxiety with the selected demographic variables of mentally ill patients in the experimental group

HYPOTHESIS

- There will be significant difference between the pre and post test scores in the level of anxiety amongmentally ill patients.

- There will be significant association between the level of anxiety and selected demographic variables

MATERIALS AND METHODS

Research approach: Quasi Experimental approach.

Research Design: Non equivalent control group pretest and post test design.

Sample Size: The sample size comprises of 60 samples

Sampling Technique: Sampling technique used for the study was purposive

sampling.Description of the Instrument

PART I: A structured questionnaire is formulated to find out the demographic

variablePART II: Hamilton Anxiety Scale was used for this study.

RESULT

The study reveals that the Experimental group the mean post test anxiety score was 20.3 .The mean post test anxiety score 4.83 of the experimental group was lesser than mean post test anxiety score 10.9 of the control group.The obtained t value 8.07 was statistically significant at 0.05 level.

Level of anxiety among mentally ill patients in experimental group

Level of Anxiety	Pre- test		Post -test	
	f	Percentage	f	Percentage
Normal(0-13)	0	-	10	33
Mild Anxiety(14-17)	2	7	16	54
Moderate Anxiety(18-24)	27	90	4	13
Severe Anxiety(25& above)	1	3	0	0

COMPARISON OF MEAN PRETEST POST TEST LEVEL OF ANXIETY OF SAMPLES IN EXPERIMENTAL GROUP

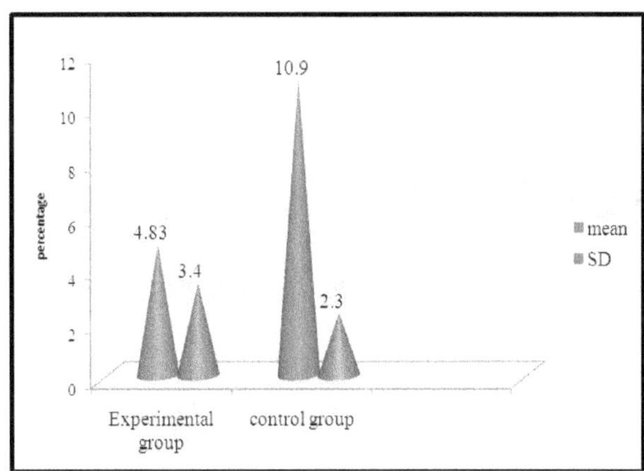

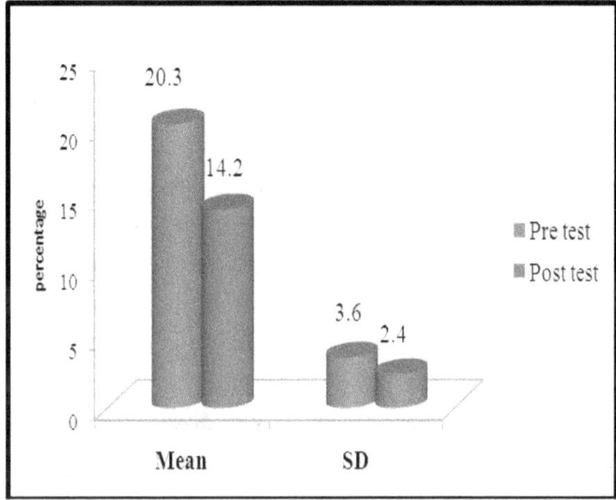

CONCLUSION

The investigator, having analyzed the data, has come to the conclusion that progressive muscle relaxation technique is an effective non pharmacologic measurement in reducing the mild and moderate levels of anxiety in chronically mentally ill patients. The investigator concludes that progressive muscle relaxation has no unpleasantness but instead it produces a pleasant effect. This can be tired in any setting of clinical practice.

REFERENCES

▣ Blazer D,(2003), "Textbook of Clinical Psychology", forth edition, New york., American psychiatry publisher.

▣ [2]. Christensen Barbara & Kockhow Elaine, (1995), "Foundation of Nursing", second edition, Philadeiphia., Lippincott Company publisher.

▣ [3]. Diahakeable, (1999), "The management of Anxiety", second edition, New York., Churchill Livingstone.

▣ [4]. Gurumani N, (2005), "An Introduction of Biostatistics", second edition, Chennai., MJP Publishers.

▣ [5]. Mary Ann Boyd, (2008), "Psychiatric Nursing Contemporary", forth edition, New Delhi., Lippincott Williams And Wilkins

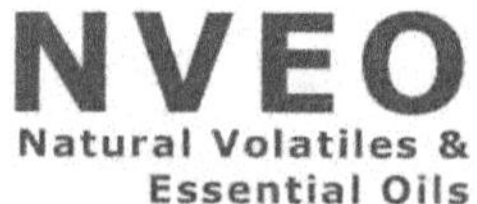

OBSESSIVE COMPULSIVE DISORDERS

¹ S.Saradhadevi, ²Dr.V.Hemavathy

¹Research Scholar, Sree Balaji College of Nursing, Bharath Institute of Higher Education and Research, Chennai,Tamil Nadu, India.
² Supervisor, Principal, Sree Balaji College of Nursing, Bharath Institute of Higher Education and Research, Chennai, Tamil Nadu, India.

Abstract

OCD is classified in the DSM-IV-TR as an anxiety disorder. It is characterized by distressing intrusive obsessive thoughts and / or repetitive actions which may be physical or mental acts that are clinically significant. Obsessive-compulsive disorder is a chronic mental illness that can have a debilitating effect on daily functioning. A body of research reveals altered sleep behavior in OCD sufferers; however, findings are inconsistent and there is no consensus on the nature of this relationship. The current study investigated whether individuals with delayed sleep phase disorder report elevated symptoms of OCD and have greater difficulty inhibiting intrusive thoughts than do individuals without Delayed sleep phase disorder. Sleep disturbances are also prevalent in obsessive-compulsive disorder as up to 48% of patients report these disturbances Previous research in OCD suggests that there is an association between specific sleep behaviors and clinical characteristics such as the severity of obsessive- symptoms, treatment resistance and age of onset of the disorder.
Keywords: OCD. Thoughts. obsessions, Anxiety

Introduction: Epidemiology

Current estimates of lifetime prevalence are generally in the range of 1.7-4%The overall prevalence ofOCD is equal in males and females symptoms usually begin in individuals aged 10-24 years,

Causes

The cause of OCD is not known; however, the following factors are relevant.

1. Genetic

2. Infections

3. Other neurological conditions :

4. Stress

5. Interpersonal relationships

OCD symptoms can interact negatively with interpersonal relationships,

Obsessions	Commonly Associated Compulsions
Fear of contamination	WASHING, CLEANING
Needed for symmetry, precise arranging	Ordering, arranging, balancing, straightening until "just right"
Unwanted sexual or aggressive thoughts or images	Checking, praying, "undoing" actions, asking for reassurance
Doubt (e.g., gas jets off doors locked)	Repeated checking behaviours
Concerns about throwing away something valuable	Hoarding

Signs and Symptoms

Common Obsessions include the Following:

- Contamination

- Safety

- Doubting one's memory or perception

- Scrupulosity (need to do the right thing fear of committing a transgression oftern religious)

- Need for order or symmetry

- Unwanted, inteusive sexual/aggressive thought

Common Compulisions include the Following:

- cleaning/washing

- checking (checking locks, stove, iron, safety of children)

- Counting/repeating actions a certain number of times or until it 'feels right'

- Arrangeing objects

- Touching/tapping objects

- Hoarding

- Confessing/seeking reassurance

- list making

Skin Findings in OCD may include the following

- Eczematous eruptions related to excessive washing

- Hair loss related to trichotillomania or compulsive hair pulling

- Excoriations related to neurodermatitis or compulsive skin picking

Treatment

1. **Pharmacotherapy**

     SSRIs (fluoxetine, filuvoxamine, sertraline, paroxetine, citalopram, escitalopram)Clomipramine , serotonin norepinephrine reuptake inhibitor (SNRI).

2. **Behavior therapy**

3. **Meditation and relation therapy**

4. **PsychotherapySurgical**

Care

- Cingulotomy or deep brain stimulation

- Transcranial magnetic stimulation (TMS)

Nursing Management

1. Try to keep them at low stress levels, especially at the start of OCD treatment.

2. Make sure that you set rigid rules for the patient's behavior and see to it that they are enforcedconsistently.

3. Encourage them to comply with behavior therapies and medication.

4. While it is a common instinct of OCD patients to seek for reassurance so as to reduce anxiety, donot allow them to indulge this habit.

5. Try to avoid comparing them with others, with or without OCD, as those with an OCD mayalready suffer from a low self-esteem.

6. Be encouraging and supportive, and help the patient set reachable goals in dealing with OCD.

Nursing Diagnosis

1. Increased Anxiety

2. Impaired coping ability

3. Altered communication pattern

4. Low self-esteem

5. Impaired Judgement

Nat. Volatiles & Essent. Oils, 2021; 8(4)

6. Self caredeficit

7. Altered sleep pattern

Bibliography

Kaj U. Koskinen, PekkaPihlantob, HannuVanharantaa Pori.2003. Tacit knowledge acquisition and sharing in a project work context. International Journal of Project Management 21 (4): 281– 290.

Dr (Mrs).K.Lalitha "Mental health and psychiatric nursing an Indian perspective" 1 st edition 2007, Page no:573-609

R.Sreevani "Mental health and psychiatric nursing" ; Jaypee brothers medical publishers(P) LTD, Page no 201-212, 240-244

KP Neeraja; "Essentials of mental health and psychiatric nursing; 2008, Jaypee brothers medical publishers ; Page no- 250

Baharuddin, Sharifah Shahnaz Syed, and Abd Hamidah Hamid. "Framing of mental health issues: A qualitative study of women's magazines in Malaysia." International Journal of Humanities and Social Sciences 3.1 (2014): 19-30.

Araujo, Flavio Soares, and Rodrigo Reboucas De Castro. "Obsessive-Compulsive Disorder: Retrospective Study on Clinical Characteristics and Family History in Outpatients Care." International Journal of Educational Science and Research (IJESR)7. 5, Oct 2017, 135-142

Devi, Luma, and V. Kavitha Kiran. "A Study on Profile and Life Style of Binge Eating People."International Journal of Educational Science and Research (IJESR) 7.4, Aug 2017, 47-52

Cáceres-Medina, Juliana, et al. "Endogenous levels of adenosine in obese patients before and after hypocaloric diet treatment." International Journal of Medicine and Pharmaceutical Sciences 5.3 (2015): 1-8.

Nat. Volatiles & Essent. Oils, 2021; 8(4)

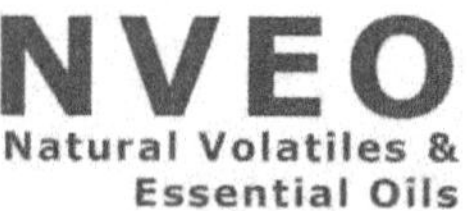

THERAPIES FOR ANXIETY DISORDERS

[1]Saradhadevi.S, [2]Dr.V.Hemavathy

[1]Research Scholar, Sree Balaji College of Nursing, Bharath Institute of Higher Education and Research [2]Supervisor, Principal, Sree Balaji College of Nursing, Bharath Institute of Higher Education and Research

Abstract

Complementary therapies are approaches to healthcare which people use as a complement to conventional care.. They are used in addition to and not instead of seeking medical advice from a doctor or taking prescribed medication.It is high quality scientific evidence of safety and effectiveness to promote health for the whole person in the context ,

Keywords: Therapy, Gestalt, Biofeedback

Humanistic Therapies
1. Person-Centred Therapy

Focuses on an individual's self worth and values. Being valued as a person, without beingjudged, can help an individual to accept who they are, and reconnect them with themselves.

2. Gestalttherapy

Is a kind of experiential therapy that emphasises personal responsibility and focuses upon the individual's experience in the present moment. The goal is to become aware of what the person doing, how he or she is doing it, and how he or she can change, and at the same time, to learn to accept and value him or herself.

By learning to follow an ongoing process, and to fully experience, accept, and appreciate the complete self, one is free to make more appropriate, spontaneous and creative contact with the environment.

3. Somatic Experiencing

Is a body-awareness approach to trauma developed by Dr. Peter Levine. Somatic experiencing restores self-regulation and returns a sense of aliveness, relaxation and wholeness to traumatizedindividuals.

4. Biofeedback

Using sensors that measure specific physiological functions—such as heart rate, breathing, and muscle tension—biofeedback teaches you to recognize the body's anxiety response and learn how to control them using relaxation techniques.

5. Hypnosis

Hypnosis is sometimes used in combination with cognitive-behavioral therapy for anxiety. While you're in a state of deep relaxation, the hypnotherapist uses different therapeutic techniques to helpyou face your fears and look at them in new ways.

Hypnosis -- or hypnotherapy -- uses guided relaxation, intense concentration, and focused attention to achieve a heightened state of awareness that is sometimes called a trance.

Hypnosis is usually considered an aid to psychotherapy (counseling or therapy) Hypnosis can be used in two ways, as suggestion therapy or for patient analysis.

- Suggestion therapy
- Analysis

OTHER TREATMENT MODALITIES FOR ANXIETY
1. COUNSELING

Psychotherapy is another type of counseling treatment for anxiety disorders. It consists of talking with a trained mental health professional, psychiatrist, psychologist, social worker, or other counselor. Sessions may be used to explore the causes of anxiety and possible ways to cope with symptoms.

ANXIETY COUNSELLING

Aims to change the patterns of behaviours, thoughts and beliefs, which trigger anxiety. De- sensitisation, which is a slow and gradual process of exposing a person to the trigger that causes anxiety to the point where the fear associated no longer poses a threat, may be used. Education about anxiety isalso an important treatment step. Anxiety management techniques are implemented which include challenging of unhelpful thoughts, learning new coping strategies, breathing exercises and relaxation training.

DEPRESSION COUNSELLING

Gives a person the skills and insight to deal with depression from a variety of angles to help prevent depression from coming back. There are many types of therapy available. Three of the more common methods used in depression include cognitive behavioral therapy, interpersonal therapy, and psychodynamic therapy. Often, a blended approach is used.

2. RELAXATION TECHNIQUES

A person who feels anxious most of the time has trouble relaxing, but knowing how to releasemuscle tension is an important anxiety treatment. Relaxation techniques include:

- Progressive muscle relaxation
- Meditation
- Abdominal breathing
- Isometric relaxation exercises.

Correct breathing Techniques

The physical symptoms of anxiety may be triggered by hyperventilation, which raises oxygen levels and reduces the amount of carbon dioxide in the blood. Carbon dioxide assists in the regulation ofthe body's reaction to anxiety and panic. A person who suffers from anxiety should learn how to breathefrom their diaphragm, rather than their chest, to safeguard against hyperventilation. The key is allowing your belly to expand as you breathe in. You can make sure you are breathing correctly by placing one hand on your lower abdomen and the other on your chest. Correct breathing means your abdomen moves, rather than your chest. It also helps to slow your breathing while feeling anxious. You can alsotry to hold your breath for a few seconds. This helps to boost carbon dioxide levels in the blood.

Exercise

Exercise is a natural stress buster and anxiety reliever. Research shows that as little as 30 minutes of exercise three to five times a week can provide significant anxiety relief. To achieve the maximum benefit, aim for at least an hour of aerobic exercise on most days.

Progressive Muscle Relaxation

A systematic technique of testing and releasing groups of muscles starting from facial muscles and moving down the body to the muscle in the feet in order to gain control over anxiety provoking thoughts and muscle tension.

3. Dietary Adjustments

The mineral magnesium helps muscle tissue to relax and a magnesium deficiency can contribute to anxiety, depression and insomnia. Inadequate intake of vitamin B and calcium can also exacerbate anxiety symptoms. Make sure your daily diet includes foods such as wholegrain cereals, leafy green vegetables and low fat dairy products. Nicotine, caffeine and stimulant drugs (such as those that containcaffeine) trigger your adrenal glands to release adrenaline, which is one of the main stress chemicals. Other foods to avoid include salt and artificial additives, such as preservatives. Choose fresh, unprocessed foods whenever possible.

4. Learning to be Assertive

Being assertive means communicating your needs, wants, feelings, beliefs and opinions to others in a direct and honest manner without intentionally hurting anyone's feelings. A person with an anxiety disorder may have trouble being assertive because they are afraid of conflict or believe they have no right to speak up. However, relating passively to others lowers self-confidence and reinforces anxiety. Learning to behave assertively is central to developing a stronger self-esteem.

5. Building Self-Esteem

People with anxiety disorder often have low self esteem. Feeling worthlessness can make the anxiety worse in many ways. It can trigger a passive style of interacting with others and foster a fear of being judged .

- Feelings of shame and guilt
- Depressed mood
- Difficulties in functioning at school, work or in social situations.

Community support organisations and counselling may help you to cope with these problems.

6. Structured Problem Solving

Some people with anxiety disorders are 'worriers', who fret about a problem rather than actively solve it. Learning how to break down a problem into its various components – and then decide on a course of action – is a valuable skill that can help manage generalised anxiety and depression.

7. Medication

It is important that medications are seen as a short-term measure, rather than the solution to anxiety disorders. Research studies have shown that psychological therapies, such as cognitive behaviour therapy, are much more effective than drugs in managing anxiety disorders in the long term. Your doctor may prescribe a brief course of tranquillisers or antidepressants to help you deal with your symptoms while other treatment options are given a chance to take effect.

Self Treatment for Anxiety

In some cases, anxiety may be treated at home, without a doctor's supervision. However, this may be limited to situations in which the duration of the anxiety is short and the cause is identified and can be eliminated or avoided. There are several exercises and actions that are recommended to cope with this type of anxiety:

- Learn to manage stress in your life. Keep an eye on pressures and deadlines, and commit to taking time away from study or work.
- Learn a variety of relaxation techniques. Information about physical relaxation methods and meditation techniques can be found in book stores and health food shops.
- Practice deep abdominal breathing. This consists of breathing in deeply and slowly through your nose, taking the air right down to your abdomen, and then breathing out slowly and gently through your mouth. Breathing deeply for too long may lead to dizziness from the extra oxygen.
- Learn to replace "negative self talk" with "coping self talk." Make a list of the negative thoughts you have, and write a list of positive, believable thoughts to replace them. Replace negative thoughts with positive ones.
- Picture yourself successfully facing and conquering a specific fear.
- Talk with a person who is supportive.
- Meditate.
- Exercise.
- Take a long, warm bath.
- Rest in a dark room.

Performance Anxiety Treatments

Here are 10 tips to help you overcome your fears and shine on stage, on the field, or at thepodium:

- Be prepared: practice, practice, practice.
- Limit caffeine and sugar intake the day of the performance. Eat a sensible meal a few hours before you are to perform so that you have energy and don't get hungry. A low-fat meal including complex carbohydrates -- whole-grain pasta, pizza, or a bean and rice burrito -- is a good choice.
- Shift the focus off of yourself and your fear to the enjoyment you are providing to the spectators. Close your eyes and imagine the audience laughing and cheering, and you feeling good.
- Don't focus on what *could* go wrong. Instead focus on the positive. Visualize your success.
- Avoid thoughts that produce self-doubt.
- Practice controlled breathing, meditation, biofeedback, and other strategies to help you relax and redirect your thoughts when they turn negative. It is best to practice some type of relaxation technique every day, regardless of whether you have a performance, so that the skill is there for you when you need it.
- Take a walk, jump up and down, shake out your muscles, or do whatever feels right to ease your anxiousfeelings before the performance.
- Connect with your audience -- smile, make eye contact, and think of them as friends.
- Act natural and be yourself.
- Exercise, eat a healthy diet, get adequate sleep, and live a healthy lifestyle.

Nat. Volatiles & Essent. Oils, 2021; 8(4)

Keep in mind that stage fright is usually worse before the performance and often goes awayonce you get started.

Treatment Modalities for Anxiety in Community

- Get out and do something you enjoy, such as going to a funny movie or taking a walk or hike.
- Plan your day. Having too much or too little to do can make you more anxious.
- Keep a diary of your symptoms. Discuss your fears with a good friend. Confiding in others sometimesrelieves stress.
- Get involved in social groups, or volunteer to help others. Being alone can make things seem worse thanthey are.
- Talk with your human resources officer about counseling benefits that may be available through your employee assistance program.
- Check with your insurance company to see what mental health benefits are available.
- Contact your public health department for information on community mental health programs.

Anxiety – Prevention

Although anxiety disorders cannot be prevented, there are ways to reduce your risk andmethods to control or lessen symptoms. Recommendations include:

- Reducing caffeine, tea, cola, and chocolate consumption.
- Checking with a doctor or pharmacist before using over-the-counter or herbal remedies to see if theycontain chemicals that may contribute to anxiety.
- Exercising regularly.
- Eating healthy foods.
- Keeping a regular sleep pattern.
- Seeking counseling and support after a traumatic or disturbing experience.
- Avoiding alcohol, cannabis.

Bibiliography

Dr (Mrs).K.Lalitha "Mental health and psychiatric nursing an Indian perspective" 1 st edition 2007, Page no: 573-609

R.Sreevani "Mental health and psychiatric nursing" ; Jaypee brothers medical publishers(P) LTD,Page no 201-212, 240-244

KP Neeraja; "Essentials of mental health and psychiatric nursing; 2008, Jaypee brothers medical publishers ; Page no- 250

Varghese, Reney, T. Selvin Norman, and Samuel Thavaraj. "Perceived stress and self efficacy among college students: A global review." International Journal of Human Resource Management and Research 5.3 (2015): 15-24.

Araujo, Flavio Soares, and Rodrigo Reboucas De Castro. "Obsessive-Compulsive Disorder: Retrospective Study on Clinical Characteristics and Family History in Outpatients Care." International Journal of Educational Science and Research (IJESR) 7. 5, Oct 2017, 135-142

Venkataraman, S., and S. Manivannan. "Mental Depression of Higher Secondary Students." International Journal of Environment, Ecology, Family and Urban Studies (IJEEFUS) 8(2018): 51-60.

Mohsin, N., W. Saeed, and H. I. Zaidy. "Comorbidity of physical disability with depression and anxiety." International Journal of Environment, Ecology, Family and Urban Studies (IJEEFUS), 3 (1) (2013).

Ababneh, Ala'A. A., Sarah M Al-Ja'freh, and Lubna Abushaikha. "Traumatic Childbirth: Incidence, Risk Factors, and Its Impact on Mothers and Their Infants a Scoping Review." International Journal of Applied and Natural Sciences (IJANS) 6.6 (2017): 1-8.

Atoum, Maysoun, and Mahmoud Alhussami. "Exploration of the Mental Health Needs and Services for Adolescents: A Qualitative Study." International Journal of Applied and Natural Sciences (IJANS) 7 (2018): 73-88.

ORIGINAL RESEARCH   Submitted: 12.04.2022; Accepted: 1.05.2022; Published online: 25.05.2022

EFFECTIVENESS OF SLEEP HYGIENE TO REDUCE INSOMNIA AMONG PERSONS WITH SUFFERING WITH OBSESSIVE COMPULSIVE DISORDER-PILOT ANALYSIS

Saradhadevi. S[1]*, V.Hemavathy

[1]Research Scholar, Department of Psychiatric Nursing, Sree Ba-laji College Of Nursing, Bharath Institute of Higher Education and Research, Chennai, Tamil Nadu
[2]Supervisor, Principal, Sree Balaji College Of Nursing, Bharath Institute Of Higher Education And Research, Chennai,Tamil Nadu

*Corresponding author: saisaradha10@gmail.com

Abstract

Obsessive-compulsive disorder frequently have insomnia, and those with acute insomnia who also have mental comorbidi- ties without therapy, they are more likely to develop persistentinsomnia. We present a case of OCD with acute insomnia that was successfully treated with early non-pharmacological sleep psychiatry intervention. Sleep is necessary for brain function and the maintenance of cognitive and emotional processes. In-somnia and anxiety problems are common, and they're linked to a lot of damage and disability. In addition to being strongly comorbid with major depressive illness, there is evidence that sleeplessness and anxiety disorders frequently co-occur. The majority of insomnia psychological therapies include sleep hy- giene. In terms of clinical practice, these instructions are a solidplace to start. Obsessive-compulsive disorder is associated withsleep difficulties. Sleep difficulties are also common in people with obsessive-compulsive disorder, with up to 48% reporting them. Obsessive compulsive disorder research reveals a link be-tween specific sleep habits and clinical factors such the severityof obsessive-compulsive symptoms, treatment resistance, and the age at which the disorder.

Keywords

Sleep, Insomnia, Obsession, Compulsion, Anxiety

Imprint

Saradhadevi. S, Hemavathy V. Effectiveness of sleep hygiene toreduce insomnia among persons with suffering with obsessive compulsive disorder-pilot analysis. Cardiometry; Issue 22; May 2022; p. 462-466; DOI: 10.18137/cardiometry.2022.22.462466;
Available from: http://www.cardiometry.net/issues/ no22-may-2022/effectiveness_sleep_hygiene_reduce

1 Introduction

Sleep disorders, particularly insomnia, are fre-quently related with psychiatric diseases, such as neu-rotic disorders, including Obsessive compulsive disor-der, which is a critical component in clinical therapy[1]. It is the inability to get the amount of sleep re-quired for optimal functioning and well-being on aregular basis a daily activity cycle that is followed [2].Going to the gym, school, and then

work, for exam-ple, is a daily cycle, whereas sitting on the couch allday and driving to the store and back is not. It's doingsomething with your body that isn't too strenuous [3].Insomnia can be short-term or long-term. Acute insomnia can persist for a few weeks or even a sin-gle night. Chronic insomnia is described as a person'sinability to sleep at least three nights per week for amonth or more. [4] ·Acute insomnia can be caused bya variety of factors, including stress, disease, physicalor mental discomfort, and a disrupted sleep cycle [5].Chronic stress, despair, and worry can all contributeto chronic sleeplessness. Insomnia can manifest itselfin a variety of ways, including difficulty falling asleep,waking up too early in the morning, and waking up inthe middle of the night and not being able to returnto sleep [6]. Yoga and meditation are two stress-re-duction strategies that might help you release energy. In addition, addressing insomnia early on can helpprevent psychiatric illnesses like depression [7]. Thelonger you wait to try to cure insomnia, the more diffi-cult it will become. Behavioral therapies for insomniainclude relaxation training, stimulus control therapy,sleep restriction therapy, sleep hygiene, paradoxicalintention therapy, cognitive restructuring, and othertechniques [8]. These are explained shortly. In personsof all ages, behavioral therapies for insomnia have beendemonstrated to be efficacious, useful, and potentially
cost-effective, with consistent, long-term results [9].

2 Review of Literature

Claudis et al. (2015) sample of 87 individuals withOCD and depression, researchers compared mind-fulness with progressive muscle relaxation provided as a bibliotherapeutic self-help technique. They found no evidence of Mindfulness's benefits in eithergroup. The programme, however, was only 6 weeks long and not therapist-led. According to Claudis etal. (2015), 47% of the respondents said Mindfulness would be more beneficial if it included interaction with a therapist.

Hamilton Fairfax* (2018) Implications for Psy- chological Intervention in Mindfulness and Obses-sive Compulsive Disorder This article summarizes themost recent research on the use of mindfulness as a treatment for Obsessive Compulsive Disorder, whichhas been a hot topic for more than a decade[3]. The application of specific models is the subject of re- search. Mindfulness and integrative treatments that incorporate Mindfulness are discussed, as well as howdescriptive components of Mindfulness may aid in understanding its role in OCD.

3 Materials and Methods

The effectiveness of sleep hygiene in reducing in-somnia among OCD people was evaluated using a quantitative evaluative research approach. The study employed an experimental research design [10]. The sample consisted of people who were addicted to alco-hol and were between the ages of 18 and 60. The prob-ability was calculated using a basic random samplingtechnique [11]. The instrument is divided into three sections: demographics, insomnia severity index scale,and interventions.

3.1. Objectives of the Study

3.1.1. To determine the pre and post assessment level of insomnia among persons suffering with obses-sive compulsive disorder in study and control group

3.1.2. To compare pre and post assessment level in-somnia among persons suffering with obsessive com-pulsive disorder in study and control group

3.1.3. To evaluate the effectiveness of sleep hygieneto reduce insomnia for persons suffering with obses-sive compulsive disorder between study and control group.

3.1.4. To associate demographic variables withposttest level of scores in study group.

4 Results

Table 1 compares the pre-intervention level of in-somnia score in the Experiment and control groups ofpeople with obsessive compulsive disorder.

Table 1

Pretest Level of Insomnia score

Level of insomnia	Experiment		Control		Chi squaretest
	N	%	n	%	
No clinically significant insomnia	0	0.00%	0	0.00%	☐2=0.37 P=0.54 (NS)
Sub threshold insomnia	1	6.67%	2	13.33%	
Moderate severity	14	93.33%	13	86.67%	
Severe	0	0.00%	0	0.00%	
C Total	15 14	100.00%	15 14	100.00%	

Before the Multi-interventional method, 6.67 per-cent of those in the Experiment group had Sub-thresh-old insomnia, while 93.33 percent had Moderate se- verity insomnia. In the control group, 13.33 percent have a score of Sub threshold insomnia, whereas 86.67percent have a score of Moderate severity [12]. Thereis no statistically significant difference. The differencebetween the Experiment and Control groups are sig- nificant. The experimental and control groups' levelsof sleeplessness were compared using the chi-square test [13].

Table 2 In the Experiment and control groups of people with insomnia, the post-test level of insomnia score obsessive compulsive disorder before interven-tion is compared in Table 2. Before the Multi-inter- ventional method, 46.67 percent of the Experiment group had Sub-threshold insomnia, whereas 53.33percent had Moderate severity insomnia.

Table 2

Posttest Level of Insomnia Score

Level of insomnia	Experiment		Control		Chi squaretest
	N	%	n	%	
No clinically significant insomnia	0	0.00%	0	0.00%	☐2=3.97 P=0.05 *(S)
Sub threshold insomnia	7	46.67%	2	13.33%	
Moderate severity	8	53.33%	13	86.67%	
Severe	0	0.00%	0	0.00%	
Total	15 14	100.00%	15 14	100.00%	

In the control group, 13.33 percent have a score of Sub threshold insomnia, whereas 86.67 percent have a score of Moderate severity. The difference between the Experiment and Control groups is statistically significant. To compare the levels of insomnia in the Ex-periment and control groups, the chi-square test was utilized.

From Table 3 In the case of the Experiment group, their pretest score was 17.93 and their posttest score was 11.40, a difference of 6.53. This difference is big and statistically significant.

Table 3

Comparison of Pretest and Posttest Mean Insomnia Score

Group		N	Mean	SD	Mean Reductio nScore	Paire dt- test
Experimen t	Pre- Tes t	15	17.93	1.2 8	6.53	t=11.55 p=0.001* **(S)
	Post- Test	15	11.40	1.2 4		
Control	Pre- Tes t	15	17.67	1.9 1	0.40	t=1.5 7 p=0.1 4(NS)
	Post- Test	15	17.27	1.0 0		

In the case of the Control group, their pretest score was 17.67 and their posttest score was 17.27, a difference of 0.40. This distinction is minor and statistically insignificant.

A student paired t-test was used to determine the difference in statistical significance between the pre- and post-test.

Taking the pretest into account, the experimental group has a 17.93 score whereas the control group has a 17.67 score, resulting in a difference of 0.93. This dif-ference is minor and statistically insignificant

From Table 4 the experimental group received a score of 11.40 on the posttest, whereas the control group had a score of 17.07, resulting in a difference of 14.57. This is a large and statistically significant difference. The statistically significant difference be- tween the experiment and the control was calculated using a student independent t-test. The pretest and posttest Insomnia scores in the Experiment and Control groups are compared using a simple bar with two standard errors.

Table 4

Comparison of Mean Insomnia Score between Experiment and Control Group

Group		N	Mean	SD	Mean Differenc eScore	Student In- dependent t-test
Experimen t		1 5	17.93	1.28	0.26	t=0.4 5 p=0.6 6(NS)
Control		1 5	17.67	1.91		
Experimen t		1 5	11.40	1.24	5.87	t=10.73 p=0.001* **(S)
Control		1 5	17.27	1.02		

The effectiveness of a multi interventional ap-proach to insomnia is shown in Table 5.

The experiment group's insomnia score was low- ered by 23.32 percent, whereas the control group's score was only reduced by 3.39 percent

The differences and generality of insomnia reduc-tion score between pretest and posttest scores were computed using the mean difference with 95 percent confidence intervals and the proportion with 95 per- cent confidence intervals.

This Table 6 illustrates association between post test level of insomnia score and persons demographic variables such as, age, religion, type of family, marital status, occupation and sleep duration and sleep habits. The relationship between the post-test level of in- somnia score and demographic factors of people is shown in Table 6. Business people/others, as well as family support people, profit more than others. The Chi square test/Yates corrected chi square test was used to determine statistical significance.

5. Discussion

Psychological and behavioral therapies with in- somnia related with medical and psychiatric illness-es, there are consistent abnormalities in various sleep metrics [14]. Sleep psychiatry (a physiologically and psychologically based psychiatric therapy meth-od based on sleep science) has gotten a lot of press around the world [15]. We sought an early interven- tion in this patient to break the vicious cycle of acute sleeplessness.

6. Conclusion

With insomnia related with medical and psychi- atric illnesses, there are consistent abnormalities in various sleep metrics. Sleep psychiatry (a physiolog- ically and psychologically based psychiatric therapy method based on sleep science) has gotten a lot of press around the world. We sought an early interven-tion in this patient to break the vicious cycle of acute sleeplessness. We hope that this study highlights the many non-pharmacological treatments that mental health professionals can utilize to treat insomnia symptoms that influence their patients' cognition, mental health, and physical well-being. Impor-tantly, re-associating the bed and bedroom with sleep-friendly behaviors, reducing sleep-incompatible behaviors, establishing a regular sleep and waking routine, and changing maladaptive thought patterns are all necessary for healing insomnia symptoms. Each of the remedies suggested has been shown to be effective in improving daily function, sleepiness, and sleep quality over time. Patients can be treated in a variety of ways, with one of the most promising being web-based administration.

Table 5

Effectiveness of Multi interventional Approach and Generalization of Insomnia reduction Score

Group	Test	Maximum score	Mean score	Mean Difference of insomnia reduction score with 95% Confidence interval	Percentage Difference of insomnia reduction score with 95% Confidence interval
Experiment	Pretest	28	17.93	6.53(5.31 –7.75)	23.32%(18.96% – 27.67%)
	Posttest	28	11.40		
Control	Pretest	28	17.67	0.40(-0.15 – 0.95)	1.42%(-0.54% –3.39%)
	Posttest	28	17.27		

Table 6

Association between Posttest Level of Insomnia Score and Persons Demographic Variables (Experiment Group)

Demographic Variables		Posttest level of Insomnia				n	Chi square test
		Sub threshold insomnia		Moderate severity			
		n	%	n	%		
Age	31-40 years	4	50.00%	4	50.00%	8	χ2=0.07p=0.78(NS)
	41-50 years	3	42.86%	4	57.14%	7	
Religion	Hindu	3	20.00%	7	80.00%	10	χ2=0.83p=0.36(NS)
	Muslim/Christian	4	100.00%	1	0.00%	5	
Type Of Family	Nuclear family	6	54.55%	5	45.45%	11	χ2=1.02p=0.31(NS)
	Joint family	1	25.00%	3	75.00%	4	
Marital Status	Married	7	46.67%	8	53.33%	15	χ2=0.00p=1.00(NS)
	Unmarried	0	0.00%	0	0.00%	0	
Occupation	Cooley /Drivers	2	20.00%	8	80.00%	10	**χ2=5.65p=0.01**(S)**
	Businessman/others	5	100.00%	0	0.00%	5	
Support System	Family	7	63.64%	4	36.36%	11	**χ2=4.77p=0.05*(S)**
	Relatives	0	0.00%	4	100.00%	4	
Duration Of Slep Per Day	2- 3 hours	1	16.67%	5	83.33%	6	χ2=1.88p=0.17NS)
	3- 4 hours	6	66.67%	3	33.33%	9	
Sleep Habits	Listing to music/others	1	16.67%	5	83.33%	6	χ2=2.88p=0.17(NS)
	Watching TV	6	66.67%	3	33.33%	9	

Statement on ethical issues

Research involving people and/or animals is in fullcompliance with current national and international ethical standards.

Conflict of interest

None declared.

Author contributions

The authors read the ICMJE criteria for authorshipand approved the final manuscript.

References

1. Segalàs C, Labad J, Salvat-Pujol N, et al. Sleep disturbances in obsessive-compulsive disorder: influ-ence of depression symptoms and trait anxiety. BMCPsychiatry. 2021; 21(1):42. Published 2021 Jan 14. doi:10.1186/s12888-021-03038-z

2. Bartleby.com was an electronic text archive, head-quartered in Los Angeles and named after Herman Melville's story "Bartleby, the Scrivener. Bartleby.com was an electronic text archive, headquartered in Los Angeles and named after Herman Melville's story "Bartleby, the Scrivener.

3. Yuichiro Abe Early Sleep Psychiatric Interventionfor Acute Insomnia: Implications from a Case of Ob-sessive-Compulsive Disorder. Published online 2012Apr 15. doi: 10.5664/jcsm.1778

4. Andrew Krystal Psychiatric disorder and sleep. HHS Public Access.Neurol clinic 2012.Nov.30(4)

5. .Katsanis et al(2014): Sleepless No More: Tech- niques and Interventions Athens Journal of Health . Volume 2, Issue 1 – Pages 9-20

6. Tenney NH, Schotte CK, Denys DA, Van MegenHJ, Westenberg HG. Assessment of DSM-IV per- sonality disorders in obsessive–compulsive disorder: comparison of clinical diagnosis, self-report question-naire, and semi-structured interview. J Pers Disord. 2003;17:550–61

7. Ruscio AM, Stein DJ, Chiu WT, Kessler RC. Theepidemiology of obsessive-compulsive disorder in the National Comorbidity Survey Replication. Mol Psy- chiatry. 2010;15(1):53–63.

8. Huppert JD, Simpson HB, Nissenson KJ, Liebow-itz MR, Foa EB. Quality of life and functional impair-ment in obsessive-compulsive disorder. Depress Anx-iety. 2009;26(1):39–45.Visser HA, van Oppen P, van Megen HJ, et al. Ob-sessive-compulsive disorder. J Affect Disord. 2014; 152–154: 169–174.

9. Eisen JL, Sibrava NJ, Boisseau CL, et al. Five-year course of obsessive-compulsive disorder. J Clin Psy-chiatry. 2013;74(3):233–239.

10. Jack D .Edinger,Behavioral and Psychological treatments for chronic insomnia disorder in adults. vol.17,2021.

11. Snehlata A. &Dwivedi,K. 2000 The effect of musican anxiety.NewDelhi Indin Psychological Abstracts and Reviews,sage Publication.

12. Mahendra P.sharma Behavioral interventions for insomnia.Indian journal of Psychaitry 2012 54(4).

13. Morin CM, Benca R.Chronic insomnia.Lance. 2012: 379: 1129-41Andrade C.Gideliness for sleepingbetter at night.Synergy Times.2004:52:

14. Ajithakumari.G.(2017). A CASE STUDY IN IN-SOMNIA. International Journal of Current Medical and Pharmaceutical Research, Vol. 3, Issue, 06, pp.1910- 1911. DOI: http://dx.doi.org/10.24327/23956429.ijc-mpr20170117

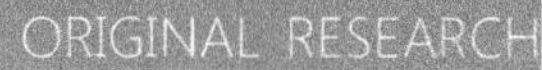 ORIGINAL RESEARCH   Submitted: 15.08.2022; Accepted: 12.09.2022; Published online: 20.11.2022

ANXIETY DISORDERS

Saradhadevi S, V.Hemavathy

Sree Balaji College of Nursing, Bharath Institute of Higher Edu-cation and Research, Chennai, Tamilnadu, India

*Corresponding author: sbcnofficialchennai@gmail.com

Abstract

Anxiety is a natural response to stress that can be beneficial in some situations. It can alert us to approaching dangers and helpus prepare and pay attention. Excessive fear or anxiety, as op- posed to usual feelings of apprehension or concern, character-ises anxiety disorders. Anxiety disorders are the most prevalentmental diseases, afflicting over one-third of the population at some time in their lives. Anxiety disorders, on the other hand, area type of mental illness. can be treated with a range of successfulmedications. The vast majority of people who receive therapy may lead normal, productive lives..It's natural to feel nervous orterrified when confronted with new, unexpected, or frighteningevents. An important test, a significant event, or a huge class pre-sentation can all create natural anxiety.. Although none of theseevents are dangerous, they may make a person feel "threatened"by potential embarrassment, Fear of making a mistake, not fittingin, tripping over words, acceptance or rejection, or loss of prideare among fears that people have. A racing heart, sweaty hands,and a jittery stomach are all physical signs of anxiety.

Keywords

Anxiety, Phobia, Obsessive ,Compulsive, Post traumatic

Imprint

Saradhadevi S, V.Hemavathy. Anxiety Disorders; Issue 24; November 2022; p. 1010-1012; DOI: 10.18137/cardiome-try.2022.24.10101012; Available from: http://www.cardiometry. net/issues/no24-november-2022/anxiety-disorders

Introduction:

Anxiety is a negative emotion marked by a state ofinternal tension as well as subjectively unpleasant sen-sations of dread about forthcoming occurrences. Ner-vous behaviour is common, including Rumination, pac-ing back and forth, and physical symptoms Worry is afeeling of unease and worry brought on by a reaction toa situation that is only seen as harmful subjectively. [1]

Symptoms include muscle tension, restlessness, fatigue,inability to catch one's breath, abdominal tightness, anddifficulty focusing. Anxiety, on the other hand, is a fear-ful reaction to the prospect of a future threat. Fear is anatural reaction to a current threat, whether genuine orimagined. Nervous people may withdraw from situa-tions that have previously made them feel unpleasant.Anxiety is a typical human reaction., but it can be clas-sified as an anxiety disorder if it is intense or lasts forlonger than developmentally appropriate intervals. [2]Anxiety disorders are classified into various categories,each with its unique clinical description (for example,Generalized Anxiety Disorder and Obsessive Com- pulsive Disorder). The fact that it is chronic, lasting 6months or longer, is one of the characteristics that dis-tinguishes it from ordinary anxiety..

DEFINITION:

An unpleasant feeling of concern or fear that is ac-companied by particular bodily symptoms is referredto as anxiety.

CLASSIFICATION

Anxiety disorders are categorised into several cat-egories: generalised Anxiety disordersAnxiety disor-ders include panic attacks, phobias, post-traumatic stress disorder, and obsessive-compulsive disorders.

EPIDEMIOLOGY

Anxiety disorders are a group of illnesses that beginbefore the age of 30 and are more common in women,persons with social issues, and those with a family his-tory of anxiety and depression. Anxietydisorders wereshown to be prevalent in 13.3% of those aged 18 to 54 years old in the United States, and 10.6% of peopleover 55 years old

SYMPTOMS

Noise sensitivity ,

Mouth is dry, and swallowing is difficult. Heartpalpitations,

agitation, tremors stomachache,Insomnia,Headache etc..

GENERALIZED ANXIETY DISORDER

- Chronic anxiety state associated with uncontrolla-ble worry.

- Patients with GAD have persistent, excessive, un- realistic worry associated with muscle tension, im- paired concentration and insomnia[3]
- Complaints of shortness of breath, palpitations andtachycardia are relatively rare .
- Alcohol abuse and dependence are common in GAD patient

RISK FACTORS

Anxiety disorders in the family, increased stress, phys-ical or mental trauma, unemployment, poverty, and drugabuse are all variables that can increase the risk of GAD.

DIAGNOSITIC EVALUATION

- GAD is diagnosed when a person has problems con-trolling exaggerated or For at least 6 months, you'vebeen experiencing excessive anxiety and worry.
- Three or more of the following symptoms accompanying the anxiety or worry for at least six months:feeling tight or restless, easily fatigued, difficultiesconcentrating, impatience, and sleep problems.

PANIC DISORDER

Panic attacks, which are separate times of intense concern and pain accompanied by a variety of physio-logical symptoms, occur often and unexpectedly., arecharacteristics of panic disorder[4].

SYMPTOMS

Heart palpitations are a common symptom of a heart attack. • Chest discomfort • Shortness of breathor discomfort • Nausea • Dizziness • Fear of death • Paresthesias • Chills or hot flushes

DIAGNOSTIC EVALUATION

- A panic attack normally lasts no more than 30 minutes and peaks in 10 minutes.
- Panic disorder is diagnosed in a patient.,when he orshe has a series of unanticipated panic attacks thatare followed by one or more of the following for atleast one month: a constant fear of future attacks
- Individuals typically feel as if they are losing con-trol or dying during an episode

.PHOBIC DISORDERSSPECIFIC PHOBIA

A specific phobia is defined as any anxiety disordercharacterised by an unjustified or irrational dread of certain objects.SOCIAL PHOBIA

Social phobia is the fear of being embarrassed or criticised in social circumstances.

SYMPTOMS

Blushing, diarrhoea, sweating, and tachycardia areall common physical signs.

AGAROPHOBIA

Agarophobia is a dread of places or events that could make panic and feel imprisoned and powerless.

SYMPTOMS

Common phobias include dread of enclosed places(clustrophobia), Fear of blood and fear of flying are two of the most common fears people have.patients with social phobia,consume alcohol another sedativeson a regular basis [5]

POST TRAUMATIC STRESS DISORDERS

Patients with anxiety, mood, and drug addiction disorders are more likely to develop further anxiety, mood, and substance addiction disorders.

SYMPTOMS :

- Nightmares
- Negative Thinking And Mood
- Unwanted Distressing Memories Of The Traumat-ic Event
- Symptoms Usually Begin Early, Within 3 MonthsOf The Traumatic Incident, But Sometimes They Begin Years Afterward.
- Symptoms must last more than a month

OBSESSIVE-COMPULSIVE DISORDER

Obsessive-compulsive disorder (OCD) is a mentalcondition marked by intrusive thoughts and obsessivebehaviours that make daily life difficult.

Fears about germs and contamination, as well as hand washing, counting motions, and so on double-checking behaviours like closing a door, are all common.

NON PHARMACOLOGICALTREATMENT

Some of the possibilities include Short-term coun-selling, stress management, psychotherapy, meditation, and exercise are all examples of psychological education..

PSYCHOLOGICAL THERAPY:

In all anxiety disorders, psychological therapies (talking therapies) are generally considered first-line treatments since they give a longer-lasting response and lower relapse than medication.

Cognitive behavioural therapy is the specialised psychotherapy with the most supporting data in anxiety disorders.

In more resistant cases, treatment may last up to 16weeks or more..

NURSES ROLE IN MANAGEMENTOF ANXIETY DISORDER:

- Reassure client of his/her safety
- Allow the client to express feelings openly.
- Teach the client and family or significant othersabout phobic reactions. Dispel any myths.
- Reassure the client that he or she can learn to decreasethe anxiety and gain control over the anxiety attacks
- Identify community resources offering specializedtreatments proven as effective
- Identify community support groups
- Use therapeutic communication, milieu therapy, promotion of self-care activities, and psychobiological and health teaching and health promotion.

CONCLUSION:

Anxiety disorders are the most frequent type of mental illness, and they usually begin before or duringadulthood. Excessive dread and anxiety, as well as per-sistent and damaging avoidance of perceived threats, are key characteristics. Anxiety disorders are character-ised by abnormalities in the brain circuits that respond to danger. Genetic variables, environmental influenc-es, and their epigenetic relationships all influence therisk of anxiety disorders. Anxiety disorders frequentlycoexist with one another, as well as with other mentaldisorders, particularly depression, and somatic disor-ders. Comorbidity usually means more severe symp- toms, a higher clinical load, and more difficult therapy.The greatest way to reduce the high burden of diseasecaused by anxiety disorders in individuals and aroundthe world is by quick, accurate disease detection and proper treatment delivery, as well as scaling up of ex-isting programmes.Anxiety disorders can be helped by a variety of psychological treatments, including re-laxation training, meditation, biofeedback, and stress management. Supportive counselling, as well as cou-ples or family therapy, can help a lot of people.

REFERENCE:

1. Benjamin JS Virginia AS," Comprehensive textbook of psychiatry :, 7 th edition, Lippincott ,pg no 1834-1846
2. R Sreevani, A text book of mental health nurs-ing, 4th edition, Jaypee publication.
3. Townsend Mary C, (2007) A Text book of psychiatry; mental health nursing, fifth edition, Jay- pee publication.
4. Manisha Gupta, A textbook of therapeutic modalities in Psychiatric Nursing,
5. Bouras N, Holt G (2007). Psychiatric and Be-havioral Disorders in Intellectual and Developmental Disabilities (2nd ed.). Cambridge University Press.
6. Beck, A. T. & Emery, G. (1985). Anxiety disor-ders and phobias: A cognitive perspective. New York: Basic Books
7. Borne, E. J. (2000). The anxiety & phobia workbook (3rd Ed.). New Harbinger Publications: Oakland, CA.
8. American Psychiatric Association (2013). Di-agnostic and Statistical Manual of Mental Disorders (Fifth ed.). Arlington, VA: American Psychiatric Pub-lishing. p. 189
9. World Health Organization (2009). Pharma- cological Treatment of Mental Disorders in Primary Health Care (PDF). Geneva. ISBN 978-92-4-154769-
10. Archived (PDF) from the original on November 20,2016.
11. Gottschalk MG, Domschke K (June 2017). "Genetics of generalized anxiety disorder and relat- ed traits". Dialogues in Clinical Neuroscience. 19 (2):159–168.
12. Barlow, D. H. (2000). Unraveling the myster-ies of anxiety and its disorders from the perspective of emotion theory. American Psychologist, 1247-1263.
13. Barlow, D. H. (2002). Anxiety and its disor- ders: The nature and treatment of anxiety and panic (2nd ed.). New York: Guilford Press.
14. Eifert, G. H., Forsyth, J. P., & Hayes, S. C. (2005). Acceptance and commitment therapy for anx-iety disorders. Oakland, CA: New Harbingers Publi- cations.
15. Anxiety self help - home treatment - WebMD.(n.d.). WebMD - Better information. Better health.. Retrieved October 11, 2011.
16. Anxiety Attacks and Anxiety Disorders: Signs, Symptoms, and Treatment. (n.d.). Helpguide.org. Re- trieved September 29, 2011